BODY ART

The ultimate form of self-expression...

by

Owen Jones

2

Copyright

Published by Megan Publishing Services
http://meganthemisconception.com

Copyright Owen Jones 2024 ©

Welcome to 'Body Art - The ultimate form of self-expression...', I hope that you will find the information in this book helpful, useful and profitable.

Not only has actual tattooing found a wider demographic, but technology has expanded the methods that can be employed to enhance our bodies. Nowadays, for example, you can get a fake tattoo that will last a couple of days for a special event. In a similar vein, women can be body-painted and the casual observer would be forgiven for not seeing a naked lady.

This doesn't work so well for men, for obvious reasons!

You can also get fake tans, hair dyes, and nail varnishes that can easily be applied at home. There are also teeth whitening, cheap wigs, and coloured contact lenses available. Not to mention cheap sunglasses and fake glasses of numerous kinds.

The ultimate form of body art is plastic surgery. Many ordinary people aspire to plastic cut, tucks and nips these days – it is not only the privilege of the rich and famous. In fact, some countries, like Thailand, offer holidays that include plastic surgery (and other forms), so that your friends will hardly recognise when you return from a month's holiday!

In fact, with all the options for body art available on a typical Western high street, no-one need look the same two days running!

The information in this ebook on various aspects of body art and related subjects, such as piercing, body painting and tattoos, is organized into 18 chapters of about 500-600 words each.

I hope that it will interest those who like to write a diary and blog, or would like to, plus webmasters who need content for their online publications.

If you have any feedback, please leave it with the company you bought this book from.

Thanks again for purchasing this ebook,

Regards,

Owen Jones

Owen Jones

Table of Contents

Body Art

White Ink Tattoos

One of the latest crazes in tattooing is the white ink tattoo. White ink tattoos are far less obtrusive than full colour or blue-black tattoos. They are a lot more subtle, if you want to have a tattoo but you do not want it to be 'in everyone's face'. Basically, a white ink tattoo looks as if the tattoo artist has written it or drawn it with white chocolate

White ink tattoos are very fashionable these days and are very unusual. Traditional blue-black tattoos often denoted membership of a club of gang. Prisoners and members of violent gangs often wear or wore crude, simple tattoos that they created with a needle and a bottle of ink.

Nowadays, many famous people, especially singers, have prominent tattoos. More girls than ever before in the West have tattoos on the base of their spine. Tribal tattoos are especially popular, although most people go for the design that they like not one with a meaning that they agree with.

In fact, tattooing is one on the oldest forms of self-decoration. Oetzi, the Ice Man, found in the Italian-Swiss Alps had tattoos and it is estimated that he lived 5,300 years ago. Tattooing is probably even older than that. In Oetzi's case, it has been suggested that the tattoo artist used ink tattoos to mark acupressure points.

Tattoos were used to denote status in the olden world - status in religion, status in life, maturity, membership of a group, and other forms of status. I once met a seventy year old Berber woman in Algeria who was covered from head to foot with a tattooed network of beautiful raised brown lines.

Her son told me that she had won a beauty contest fifty years ago and that part of the prize was the red ink tattoo, because then everyone would know for the rest of her life that at one time she was the most beautiful woman in the area.

In Thailand many older men have large tattoos on their chest and their back 'to stop bullets and other weapons'. The belief that ink tattoos can confer good luck or protection from evil is one of the main reasons for tribal tattoos. They also showed membership of a group.

The white ink tattoo is the most recent development in this tradition. A white ink tattoo on a pale skinned person is barely visible. It looks like a raised layer of skin - a scar. However, a white ink tattoo on a dark-skinned person can look like white chocolate writing on a dark-chocolate birthday cake, which is very unusual and very effective.

A popular body art white ink tattoo looks like a network of beautiful Gothic scars. A light, milky white tattoo also looks good as a wrist tattoo or a hand tattoo.

Barcode Ta too

The barcode tattoo is another recent style development in the ever-evolving world of body art. The barcode tattoo is a symbol of the modern world we live in, but could be quite useful if the barcode tattoo gave your name, social security number and blood group. If you were ever involved in a serious accident, your barcode tattoo could save your life, if it is somewhere prominent like your wrist or hand.

Tattooed Eyebrows

Body art and facial tattoos, including tattooed eyebrows are also fashionable. Maybe it has something to do with Star Trek! Some women use very subtle tattooing on their eyes as a form of permanent mascara. My wife has tattooed eyebrows. They stand out as being unusual for a few months, but later fade and blend into the face becoming less obtrusive. Or maybe I have just become accustomed to her tattooed eyebrows.

Anchor Tattoos

Anchor tattoos are some of the oldest tattoos. Sailors and other sea-faring folk used representations of the anchor to symbolize hope and stability. Popeye the Sailor man has an anchor tattoo on his upper arm. An anchor on a traditional Welsh Love Spoon meant: 'I am home forever'. If you like anchor tattoos, think about what an anchor means to someone in a small boat on the sea.

Men's Tattoos

There used to be a definite line where you could say, these are men's tattoos and these are women's tattoos, but these distinctions are blurring. Anchor tattoos are traditionally men's tattoos because there were not many women sailors. Women preferred ephemeral tattoos - patterns, butterflies and flowers. Dragon tattoos were also traditionally men's tattoos, but women wear them too nowadays.

Barcode Tattoos

The barcode tattoo is one of the more modern custom tattoos. However, there are problems with the typical bar code tattoo that are not immediately apparent. They look like something out of a science fiction story. To start with, barcode scanners are made to read quite precise codes and not all barcode tattoos are drawn accurately enough to be scanned. This is not the only potential problem with your lovely barcode tattoo though

Most people are interested in having a barcode tattoo as a custom barcode memento of their personal details such as name, national security number or and blood type. There is plenty of software available that will transform your personal details into a barcode.

That is the least of your problems. if you are not worried about a personalized, readable barcode then you can get a standard image from a catalogue or use a temporary body decal bar code tattoo.

The biggest problem with a barcode tattoo is 'creep'. A barcode consists of vertical black or blue lines on a grid that can take 95 vertical lines. These lines are quite close together, so as a tattoo blurs with age, it becomes impossible for a barcode reader to read your barcode tattoo any longer.

If the tattoo is too small, the lines of ink run into each other over time, which is quite normal. This happens with all tattoos sooner or later depending on several factors such as where they are on the human body and how old the wearer is and what condition he or she is in.

There are a few things you can try to overcome this natural phenomenon, but most tattoo artists are not aware of the problem or do not understand how to prevent it. The first thing to try is to enlarge the tattoo a little. Most barcode tattoos are one-and-a-half to two inches wide, which is the standard commercial size.

The problem is that this size barcode tattoo will blur quite quickly. The tattoo artist should stretch the barcode tattoo to two-and-a-half inches wide. However, making the tattoo wider than that will probably render it unreadable to most scanners, because the beam is only accurate to 2.5" wide.

The other thing that the tattoo artist, in conjunction with the customer, can do is locate the tattoo on an area of skin that does not stretch or sag too much. Flat, taut areas of the human body that do not have much fat under them are the best. Therefore, the wrist, the foot, the ankle or calf and the back are the best.

It is best to avoid 'fatty' or muscular areas like the upper arm and the neck for barcode artwork, unless you are using a temporary body decal bar code.

Some people place their barcode tattoo on their ear or temple, which normally works well enough for the young, although the ear is not really large enough or flat enough to take a permanent readable barcode.

Who would have thought that so much science would go into getting a simple, readable barcode tattoo?

Body Art

Tattooed Eyebrows

Tattooed eyebrows are a form of permanent make-up. Some women like to have a professional make-up artist do a first class job of their eye make-up and then have it permanently tattooed onto the eye area. If done properly, tattooed eyebrows ensure perfect eye make-up 24 hours a day, without the risk of it spoiling.

Professional swimmers and actresses like some form of eyebrow tattoo. Actresses may prefer less than the full make up so that they can be more flexible, but professional athletes, especially swimmers and divers, tend to go for professionally shaped brows permanently tattooed on.

In fact, this form of tattooing is nothing new. There are two types of eye tattooing: permanent and semi permanent. Permanent eyebrows do not need to be touched up from time to time whereas the semi permanent makeup method does. Although this form of cosmetic tattooing is not new, it is only just catching on with the general public.

Many women who go for permanent make-up also have tattooed eyeliner and lip liner implanted to help show off their eyebrow arches and bone structure. The colour is implanted with a normal tattoo needle gun and hurts just as much (or not) as normal tattooing too.

The technical difference between the two types of tattoo is that the semi permanent eyebrows tattoos are placed on top of the skin, whereas the permanent kind is a straight forward tattoo where the colour is implanted as in normal tattooing.

The beauty of having tattooed eyebrows or any other facial cosmetic tattoo is its permanence. If a woman leads a hectic lifestyle, tattooed eyebrows will save quite a bit of time over a month. Similarly with eyeliner tattooing and lip liner. She will be beautiful 24 hours a day

It is not only the saving in time, it also allows the tattooed person to go swimming or build up a sweat without a chance of the 'makeup' running, which is very useful for people who enjoy jogging or working out in public places like a gymnasium.

The art of eyebrow tattooing probably started in the East either in Japan, where it has been popular for hundreds of years or in Polynesia where Captain Cook's expedition discovered 'tatau' among the islanders. The islanders used a lot of cosmetic tattoo makeup on their faces.

The make-up artist or tattoo artist who is responsible for tattooing your eyebrows has a wide range of colours to choose from these days, so you can either choose your natural colour or pick one that you prefer.

If you are unsure which colour tattoo make up you should have, the tattoo artist can advise you, but it is probably better to try a temporary eyebrow tattoo first. If you do not like the colour, you can change it next time until you et it right.

Most tattoo artists that do eyebrow tattoos also have a range of pictures of tattooed eyebrows to help individuals make up their minds exactly what semi-permanent makeup to tattoo on.

I am assured by my wife that permanent tattooing on your eyebrows is not very painful after the first three or four hours, and that semi permanent makeup tattooed eyebrows do not hurt at all.

Body Art

Men's Tattoos

In the West, until about 40-50 years ago, only men wore tattoos. The most common forms of mins tattoos were the sword or dagger for soldiers and the anchor for sailors. Women still do not wear these symbols often as they are considered mins tattoos. Women tend to go for symbols with 'nicer' meanings, although the anchor tattoo is becoming fairly common with women too.

In fact, the lines of demarcation between women's and men's tattoos is blurring. For example, a woman might not wear traditional Celtic designs, but she will wear modern Celtic tattoos with modern Celtic designs: flowers, trees, dragons, Celtic crosses and hearts.

It should not be forgotten that the original reason for most wearing tattoos was aggressive. Warriors wore tattoos into battle to frighten their enemies and ward off bad luck - two aggressive actions. The tradition passed into the Royal Navy and from there to most of the navies in the world.

Members of the armed forces all over the world often wear tattoos too. This is why there is a class of tattoos that could be referred to as mins tattoos -

they tend to be the more traditional styles. You must have seen a dagger on a soldier's forearm or upper arm with blood and 'Death or Glory' written on it.

Surely, you have seen the beautiful Lady Luck, often naked, in the same locations or the Popeye the Sailor style anchor tattoo? Mins tattoos are usually displayed more prominently than those on women, which are usually hidden in discrete, personal places on the body. Men often have forearm tattoos and tattoos on the upper arm.

However, if you are wondering which design to have tattooed on you, remember that the ultimate choice is yours alone. if you want a few flowers on your ankle, why not? However, most men go for the more traditional mins tattoo designs. If you want to go down that route too either ask the tattoo artist for a catalogue of ideas for men to choose from or download what you want from a site like those you will find on this website.

There are plenty of cool tattoo designs for men: look at the dragon tattoos and the Celtic or religious tattoos. Tribal arm tattoos are very popular on the upper arm or forearm. Tribal tattoos are often seen on as leg tattoos or upper back tattoos as well.

Look around and you will find lots of tattoo ideas for men.

How about a skull tattoo or a neck tattoo? They are very popular with men but far less so with women. Eagle tattoos are very popular with American men, while men from other countries might also like birds of prey, lions, tigers or snakes. Dragon tattoos too.

The back is a great place to have these done because the area of skin is so large. Upper back tattoo designs are really impressive on men, as lower back tattoo designs are on women.

There is only one thing to bear in mind when choosing mins tattoos as far as I can see: if you pick it out of the tattoo artist's catalogue, so have dozens of others probably, so why not get your own tattoo design and take it to the tattoo artist for a quote?

This is the only real way to ensure that you get tattooed with unique men's tattoos. However, you could always try a few fake tattoos until you find one you like.

Body Art

22

Trends in Jewellery

There are trends in jewellery as much as there are trends in clothes, shoes and colours. However, because jewellery is such an old concept, there are classic designs that are always popular because they always have been. Grandparents tend to hand this type of classic jewellery down, while people tend to buy the current trends in jewellery.

It is virtually impossible for the average person to guess what the next trend will be, but there still things that you can do, which we will look at later in this piece. First, we will define some of the areas that are affected in trends in jewellery

People tend to wear different types of jewellery in the day to in the evening; at work to on holiday; in their youth than in their more advanced years and perhaps even in the summer to in the winter. If you do not adopt some kind of tactic towards trends in jewellery, it can get very expensive indeed.

Daytime jewellery can be bright, cheerful and fairly cheap. Large earrings, a large, loose necklace of beads of wood, plastic or glass and matching large bracelets are fine. They brighten the day and if you lose something or a child breaks something, it is not so important. holiday jewellery can or even should be more fun still and cheap is the order of the day as you lie on the beach or by the pool.

Jewellery at work should probably trend more towards the classic, but it can depend on your job. If you meet clients, a dress code is more important than if you work in the back office. Working in a factory also affects the jewellery that you wear. The last thing that you want is to get it caught in a machine. Even rings are dangerous at work.

Evening wear should also be classical. There is not a lot of trending in evening jewellery This is especially true of people who feel unsure of themselves in a formal situation. Everyone knows that classic is always suitable, in the same way that the black dress or dark suit is always acceptable. It takes courage to stand out from the crowd.

If you have a collection of jewellery, the way to stay looking trendy is with accessories. By this people normally mean: bags, purses, head wear and scarves. It is just as good to have a large collection of costume jewellery and accessories when trying to follow the trends in jewellery

If any long term trend in jewellery is discernible, it is that people are turning away from traditional jewellery like gold and diamonds, which they see as over priced. This is a good thing as you do not need to spend hundreds on a tiny diamond mounted in 9 or 14 carat gold, when you could get a beautiful turquoise or citrine for a quarter of the price.

The best tip is to trust your own judgment and let your own fashion style shine through. Show or start your own trend in jewellery today.

Body Art

Professional Teeth Whitening

"Smile and the world smiles with you", so they say and there is no doubt that a beautiful smile is infectious. So, how do you get a beautiful smile if you smoke, drink coffee or red wine or like curry? Age affects the colour and staining of your teeth too as can illness and medication. Lifestyle and attitude also play part in having and maintaining a lovely, whiter smile.

You could try home tooth whitening, but it takes time and sustained effort over weeks or even months. If you do not think you could keep that up, you should try a professional light activated tooth whitening treatment by a dentist.

Professional teeth whitening is a technique by which whitening compounds that are peroxide (hydrogen or carbamide) based are applied to teeth by dentists within their dental office. Laser teeth whitening is the common practice of dentist to whiten teeth stained by nicotine, food, or dark liquids.

Peroxide-based whitening compounds usually depend on two factors:

1. The concentration of peroxide in professional teeth whitening products

2. The amount of time a whitener is put in contact in the surface of the teeth Laser teeth whitening utilizes a higher concentration of whitener for a shorter period of time, say for hours or for a few appointments.

The whitening compounds and associated equipment (bleaching light or laser) used by dentists are normally purchased from a manufacturer as a franchise, system, or simply as a kit. In fact, many manufacturers have provided national campaigns about their whitening products and equipment.

Dentists play a vital part in the promotion of a manufacturer's cosmetic product because they are actually using the product on their patients.

Below is a list of some professional whitening products dentists and professionals choose. (The kind of bleaching laser or light is enclosed in parentheses.)

1. BriteSmile (gas plasma light/light emitting diode) 2. LaserSmile (a Biolase laser) 3. LumaArch (halogen light) 4. Rembrandt Sapphire (plasma arc light) 5. Zoom! (metal halide light)

Each of these whitening systems has its own degree of effectiveness. However, we can summarize three standard steps when using these types of products.

1. The dentist will compare the tooth shade of the patient with a tooth shade guide. Surface stain and

tartar are removed before determining the tooth shade. A dentist needs to document a pre-treatment and a post-treatment tooth shade to assess the effectiveness of the whitening treatment system applied.

A dentist may make use of variously shaded tooth-shaped porcelain tabs and compare them to a patient's set of teeth and each match is documented. Some dentists even take pictures of a patient's teeth before and after the treatment. Flour of pumice is used to polish each tooth to ensure that stains are completely removed.

2. The dentist will isolate teeth being whitened. Bleaching agents, normally peroxide-based, can irritate or even damage delicate tissues within the mouth of patients. To protect these tissues, dentist use dental dam barriers. Thin sheet of latex punched with a hole for each tooth and dental gels painted around each tooth are used to protect the teeth being treated.

When the latter is used, a cheek retractor, cotton rolls and gauze are used to make sure that the patient's lips and cheeks are held out of the way. Afterwards, these items are simply peeled off.

3. Bib covering and eye protection are placed on the patient. Unexpected things can happen. Bibs are worn by patients to protect their skin against the caustic nature of these bleaching agents. Eye protection is also placed to ensure that whiteners will not irritate even the eyes of the patients.

Moreover, it is a common knowledge that an intense bleaching light or a laser used to activate the components of bleaching compounds could cause eye damage.

What else can I do if I have undergone professional whitening?

To get rid off typical stains of the coffee and cigarette variety, they can be washed away alternately with professional tooth whitening systems. Here are some additional tips: Munch some apple and drink water afterwards.

Brush after every meal to have a less chance of keeping stains on your teeth. Brush gently but effectively by using a dentist-approved toothpaste and toothbrush. Practice the correct ways of brushing.

Researchers on dentistry note that an electric toothbrush removes over 95% of plaque. Gargle with a mouthwash that has an antibacterial action. This practice will surely will reduce stain-catching plaque.

Don't depend on quick-fix remedies like using super-whitening tooth polishes because these also make the enamel of teeth thinner. And as enamel gets thinner, more of the dentin will show off making your teeth appear heavily stained.

To put it simply, here are some reasons why or why not to choose professional teeth whitening products.

1. The effect can be seen instantly.

2. The whitening can be completed in just a few appointments (possibly even just one).

3. Professional tooth whitening remedies cost more than do-it-yourself teeth whitening treatments.

Body Art

32

Push Up Bikinis

Who has not wanted to look bigger, if you are smaller? That is why the Playtex bra was invented and the push up bikini is just a flattering extension (no pun intended) of the same idea. There are several ways of designing push up bikinis and really it is up to the wearer to find out what is best for her. Just as with bras. But do not forget that many women wear the wrong size bra for themselves. If you want a push-up bikini, it would be worth asking the assistant's advice.

The first bikini like garments that we know of are depicted in a mosaic dating back to about 300 BC. It shows ten young women exercising in what we would recognize as triangle top bikinis. The bikini did not have a revival in the West until the modern bikini was 'invented' in 1946 by a French engineer.

A bikini is really a set of modern women's underwear, which looks great and natural and is acceptable as beachwear. The top has the same function as a brassiere and the bikini bottom functions as panties. Therefore, you could say that the technology that is used is bras is also being used in bikini tops and one of the features that a lot of women like in bras is the push up effect, which you can now see in the underwire swimsuit.

Push up bras are usually designed just to give a woman a more prominent bust line, but a push-up bikini is also meant to enhance a woman's cleavage, which is normally covered by a blouse in everyday female clothing. Most women who favour push up bikinis are younger women in their first years of wearing sexy bathing suits and women with a smaller bust.

Support and lift can be provided by push up bikinis using several methods. The cups may be supported by under-wiring or not. The under-wiring can become hot, so some manufacturers coat the wire in plastic.

Strapless push up bikinis usually have to use some form of under-wiring although there are wire free strapless bikini tops which do their job by making use of larger cups and wider straps. This latter type are often referred to as soft cup push-up bikinis.

Many bikinis that are meant to enhance the breasts have comfortable, flattering padding, but this padding can also serve to hide the nipples of modest ladies, especially when swimming in cold water.

Many women wear bras and bikinis that are not quite suitable for them, so it is wise to get an expert to help you choose the right size, especially if you have just lost weight or are still growing.

Some larger busted women also want to wear push up bikinis and the way these women usually solve the questions of support and lift is to use a halter with fairly large triangles of fabric to provide two separate cups. Under-wired swimsuit push up bikinis frequently only go up to size D cup.

However, from a man's perspective, what most women who wear push up swimwear seem to forget is that women in a bikini are almost naked already so they do not really need to do a lot more than that!

Body Art

Anchor Tattoos

People associate anchor tattoos with sailors and that is hardly surprising, but anchor tattoos are also popular with non-sailors these days and that is because there are stunning anchor designs and the anchor has come to symbolize hope and stability. The anchor tattoo is definitely one of the best developed tattoos because it has been around so long.

Anchor tattoos were the first tattoo design to become popular in the West and that was among sailors. The concept of the tattoo was originally 'rediscovered' by Captain Cook in the mid-Eighteenth century on the island of Samoa and so it was natural for those sailors to tattoo themselves with symbols of the items that were around them every day.

Anchors and ships, beautiful ladies (OK, only in port, but definitely on their minds), symbols of good luck and mementos of home were all very common among sailors and the practice spread from the British merchant and royal navies to other navies around Europe and, from there, the world.

It has been said that early Christians used the anchor symbol instead of the cross tattoo because they are similar, but displaying the cross in early Christianity dominated by Roman pagans meant death or persecution. This is probably also true.

In modern times, US sailors use the anchor tattoo to mark a right of passage. It means that they have been across the Atlantic and come back home again by sea. This is a symbolism unique to American sailors as far as I can determine. Sailors from other countries do not need a reason to wear the anchor tattoo.

The anchor tattoo has also been used to imply that the wearer is happy with someone. For example, during the Second World War, it was very common for young sailors in the Royal Navy or the Merchant Navy to have an anchor tattoo with 'Mum and Dad' written across it, because many of those young lads had never had a girlfriend, whose name they could have put there instead.

These old tattoos were never really popular with people who had no connection with the sea, but that is changing now. There is a huge demand for things retro and anchor tattoos fall into this category. Men and women, who have never even been on a boat are getting anchor tattoos now.

They do not wear the anchor tattoo as a sign that they have worked at sea or made specific voyages, they wear them for their symbolism of safety, being 'at home' (with someone) and good luck, which is similar to its meaning on the old Welsh love spoons.

However, one of the biggest, latest trendy tattoos is white ink tattooing and one of the most popular of them is the white ink anchor tattoo. The white ink anchor tattoo is basically an update of the old style anchor tattoo. Retro often has a habit of slightly changing the old style.

In the case of white ink anchor tattoos, it is the white ink, because old style anchor tattoos would have been in blue or black possibly with a little red, but modern all white ink anchor tattoos are something stylish and very, very different. White ink tattoos are definitely here to stay.

Body Art

40

Tattoo Designs

If you have never been into a tattoo artist's studio, you would probably be quite astonished. Tattooing has a very sleazy reputation, but that is because of its association previously with tattooists on the dock or in prison. It is nothing like that any more. They are professional, clean and hygienic. Tattooists are called tattoo artists and their places of business are called tattoo studios, like artists' studios.

This is because the majority of tattoo artists are artists in their own right. They can frequently draw on other surfaces than human skin as well. Lots of them can paint or draw on canvas or paper. However, most customers prefer to either look through the tattooist's catalogue of images or go to a web site from which they can download a picture of their choice.

There are more types of tattoos online and that means that there is less chance that you will meet people with the same tattoo designs on the bodies. This is especially true if you want popular tattoo designs such as a dragon, dragonfly, butterfly, tiger, snake, skull. heart, eagle, wolf or rose.

This can be a big thing if you like to stand out from the crowd or an image has a personal significance to you.

Some web sites have as many as 10,000 traditional and modern images. In fact, going on line is probably the best way of procuring your tattoo picture, because the old ones are being redesigned all the time adding new twists to traditional tattoo designs.

But, if you choose from a tattoo studio's catalogue, you will almost certainly see your tattoo on someone else as well, whereas if you download one from the Internet, the chances of seeing it on someone else are far smaller.

However, if you go to a decent tattooist, you need just describe what you want and it will be copied to your skin, because the best tattooists are also artists, as was pointed out above.

Having said that, some individuals like to have duplicate tattoo designs, because the picture has been made well-known by a celebrity. Besides the celebrity look-alike copies there are also numerous tribal tattoos. Millions of people all around the world have copied their screen idols' tattoo designs.

Traditional tattoo designs from cultures across the world are fashionable. Native American artwork is very popular in North America and Thai and Korean traditional tattoo designs are popular everywhere, not only in their home countries.

Other notable, commonplace tattoos denote membership of a club or a gang. For instance, numerous men who have spent time in Cardiff Prison tattoo themselves with the image of a bluebird on their thumb, but the bluebird is also the emblem of Cardiff City Football Club. The tattoo may also be found frequently on the neck.

Sailors also (used to) sport tattoo designs to denote their occupation or as a guard against bad luck or the perils of the deep.

Signs of the Zodiac are also fairly universal and the zodiacal images are quite standardized, but the likelihood of seeing yours on someone else is far less that one-in-twelve. Dragons are also ubiquitous even if it is only on the skin. At one time, dragon tattoos were just worn by men, but these days women wear them almost as frequently

Religious and Celtic symbols are very common too. Crosses, Celtic Crosses, Jesus on the Cross and others can be seen frequently. Then there are the tattoos that are more the province of women, but not exclusively so. These include complex designs, flowers, birds, dolphins, butterflies and cherries.

It is a good thing that the lines between what are male and what are female tattoos are blurring, but they have not yet disappeared totally by any means. Not many women wear tattoos of anchors, knives, 'LOVE and HATE', 'MUM and DAD' on their knuckles or naked men on their arms, but who knows, it may yet come, or not?

Body Art

Tattoos around the World

Oetzi, the Iceman found in the Swiss-Italian Alps, was a traveller. No-one lived up there in those freezing conditions, so he must have been going from one place to another. He was a traveller, possibly an outcast. He lived 5,300 years ago and he had 53 tattoos. The marks are still clearly visible on his parchment-like skin. it has been suggested that the purpose of some of the tattoos was to mark pressure points for acupuncture or other medicinal purposes.

The Celts of Europe and particularly those of Britain were renowned for their use of bodily and facial tattoos. Briton actually means 'people of the designs' and the Scottish Picts were the 'painted people'. The British are still the most tattooed individuals in Europe. How's that for tradition living on throughout history?

Tattooing is an ancient form of body art, although it almost certainly had either religious connotations or connections with showing rank and status. Tattooing has to have travelled with travelling people.

Tattooing must have spread all over the globe, wherever man went trading. Sailors are, or at least were, very superstitious people and sailors the world over are renowned for their tattoos.

In some cultures, traditionally the most beautiful girls and women were tattooed to prove for the rest of their lives that they were once of exceptional beauty. it is considered a boost in status.

Despite, let's guess, 5,500 years of a tattooing tradition, it is only now becoming acceptable in 'polite society' in the West thanks mainly to film stars, pop idols and sports personalities, but how do people in other parts of the world regard tattoos? In the West, they are almost purely ornamental now, but do other countries with different cultures have other uses for them still?

Some countries, Eastern and Western, used to brand or tattoo criminals, so these people used to try to keep their tattoos covered up after they were released from prison. In the Fifteenth Century condemned men were tattooed with a rose so that if they escaped they could easily be recognized. These men would definitely have covered their tattoo.

However, the history of tattooing criminals (and slaves) goes back much further than that. Romans used tattoos to identify their troops, their slaves and their gladiators. British (ex-pat) and American slave-owners used tattoos to identify their slaves and even tattooed them 'Tax Paid'.

Romans tattooed the faces (foreheads) of slaves with 'Stop me I am a runaway'. The Nazis tattooed the forearms of concentration camp prisoners with their ID number both to identify them and to embarrass them as tattooing goes against the Jewish religion.

Tattooing in its contemporary Western variety comes from the Polynesian islands and was transported back to Britain by the English explorer Captain Cook and his sailors in the Eighteen Century. It was called tatau, but the word steadily became anglicized and spread throughout Europe among the seafarers, sailors and explorers.

Tattoos are associated with violence in many countries. Tattooing in Japan, especially full or very large body tattoos are used to identify members of the different Yakuza (mafia) gangs. The Russian mafia uses them too.

A 2004 survey in Britain revealed that 72% of those surveyed with head, neck or hand tattoos had spent at least three days in jail in comparison with 6% of the non-tattooed populace.

The Latin word for 'tattoo' is 'stigma' from which

we get the word 'stigmatize', which gives an accurate impression of what European societies in general think about tattoos. In other countries, such as Thailand, Laos and Cambodia, tattoos are frequently used to ward of bad luck and attract good luck.

Upper-Body Art

The human upper body, especially the back, makes an ideal canvas for all forms of body art including tattooing and body painting. If you are considering your first upper-body artwork, you could do worse than have it be an upper back tattoo. You could put your art and soul into it!

Upper back tattoos can range from small and simple to large and elaborate, and can stand alone or be the foundations for larger and more elaborate personalised and custom tattooing, if you like the outcome and want to add to it. Upper back tattoos are, more often than not, covered in indoor settings so they won't be an issue in professional environments.

Women considering upper back tattoos will have to decide if their social life is a deterrent; backless formal gowns. You may consider them to be unwearable once upper-body art has been applied to it. But a small tasteful tattoo has found its way to many a female celebrity's upper back, so the bias against female tattoos in upper social circles may be fading. Tank tops and bating suits will also be a giveaway for upper-body art and tattoos, but in the casual environment at the poolside they are not only accepted; they are often admired.

Any upper-back tattoos you are considering should be a topic of conversation between you and your tattoo artist before you make any decisions. Placement is key, so that you can incorporate your design into a later full back tattoo if you so desire. At the same time, you don't want your upper-back tattoo to be so oddly positioned that it sticks out like a sore thumb.

You'll also have to consider the amount of time you are accustomed to spending shirtless in the sun. You should be using sunscreen anyway, even if you don't have tattoos, but sun exposure is a big contributor to the fading of body art and tattoos. Your upper back tattoo is going to fade, because that is what tattoos do, but there's no reason for you to speed the process simply because you forgot the sunscreen.

One big positive to having an upper-back tattoo as your first is that they are much less prone to infection than tattoos in other areas. However, you'll still be responsible for following your tattoo artist's after-care safety directions, which will include periods of exposing your tattoo to the air to help it dry. So, consider the time of year when you get your tattoo. Being topless in January in your part of the world might be cold.

Nicolas Cage with a monitor lizard wearing a top hat; David Beckham with his son's name above a Crucifixion scene; LeBron James with Chosen 1; Fabio Cannovaro with his daughter's name; Melanie Chisholm with a phoenix; and Laura Headley, with a lotus blossom, are just a some of the many celebrities who have chosen upper-back tattoos to say something about themselves or the things that matter to them.

If you do an online search for upper-body tattoo or painting designs, you're sure to be amazed at the variety of designs from small and simple to incredibly intricate, and somewhere among them find the one which is just right for your taste.

Body Art

52

Body Painting

These days, the most common forms of body art are tattooing and body piercing, but human body painting is also popular with certain groups of people. Face painting is very common among children and followers of sports teams. Actual full-body artwork is usually restricted to female models, since it is far more difficult to design an image which will camouflage the male genitalia and it is not acceptable to display those parts in public.

Two of the most common forms of total body paintings is to paint sports kits and swimsuits onto nude female models, so that from a distance or from certain angles, it looks as if the women are wearing sports clothing. There have been many photographs of such female models in the body art in the press, so I am sure you have seen them too.

These days world body painting festivals are commonplace and bring national and international Body Painting Awards. If you are interested in these body art festivals, search on the Internet to find out when the next one is nearest to where you live. They are useful if you want to pick up experience in body art, the latest techniques, or just materials.

Face and body painting is a form of body art, and has almost certainly been around since the beginning of civilization. In almost every tribal culture, body painting was performed during ceremonies or merely just for the beauty of it. Often, body painting had a spiritual significance and the natives of many countries, including the British Isles, America, Canada, and Australia used body painting and face painting for protection from their enemies and wild animals.

The ancient British, the Celts, used woad as a blue body paint and war paint was common in many countries. Back then they used clay and other natural pigments. Painting the skin of a person still survives in most parts of the world, especially Mehndi, which is the form that uses henna dyes. It is now very popular in the western world too. The henna tattoo is semi-permanent. Since the 1960's, body painting has emerged as an actual art form. However, there is the never-ending discussion about it's social acceptability because body painting practically always involves total nudity.

However, no art without paint of course, and you'll be happy to know that the paint is restricted by guidelines: the body paint has to be non-toxic and non-allergenic. The paint easily washes off with water and soap. As for the henna dyes, which Mehndi uses, there's a difference between the synthetic black henna, and the natural brown henna. The natural henna dye is completely safe when body painting, but the synthetic black henna dye could cause allergic reactions. You should have yourself patch tested before using these at body painting.

Besides nudity, which is less of an issue these days, body painting is not without controversy, which you might say has always been the case in the art world. This aspect of body painting is outside the scope of this piece, however, you might like to look up the names of Rebecca Horn, Youri Messen-Jaschin, Javier Perez, Marina Abramović and Jana Sterbak.

Body Art

Gold Earrings

Gold is a very unusual commodity, isn't it? It has been in high demand in most of the world since time immemorial. In that respect it is timeless. It has a strange allure, yes, it is rare and so expensive, but seems to go deeper than that. Gold has almost a religious significance. Think of the golden robes of some monks or the golden halos painted above saints' heads.

Most people want to own some .gold, if not for its monetary value, for the style and elegance that it imbues the wearer with. Gold jewellery goes will all or no clothes - you can wear it with the most formal clothing imaginable or in your birthday suit and it looks just as good. That cannot be said for anything else except diamonds, so it is not surprising that diamonds are often mounted in an item of gold.

Perhaps the simplest jewellery of all are the stud or hoop earrings. Most women, even the poorest, strive to possess a set of gold earrings. Most teenage girls want to have their ears pierced to receive such earrings and in some cultures, ear piercing is part of growing up - especially in Asia. Gold is the ideal metal to be in contact with sensitive body parts because it is completely inert.

Pure gold will never tarnish, so it cannot cause a reaction. However, gold is really sold pure on the jewellery market because it is too soft to be worn regularly. Pure it is too malleable, it bends and beaks. The clasp would be unreliable, so an expensive item could easily drop off and be lost. Even stud earrings work loose and fall out.

When buying gold earrings, or any item for that matter, you should be concerned about its purity or quality - how much gold is actually in the items. We already know that it has to be mixed into an alloy, but with what and to what percentage? The gauge is called the carat or carat often shortened to kt. or ct. The higher the number, the purer the gold.

24 carat is pure gold, but is not used in jewellery. Not all countries use the carat yardstick, some use a percentage. Therefore, 24ct is 100%; 18ct is 75%; 12ct is 50% and so on. The highest value of carat used for jewellery is 22ct with 18ct being more usual. Then 14ct is common and 9ct is the lowest used, although it is only 37.5% gold.

People talk of white gold, yellow gold, red, pink and rose gold, but gold is gold and it is yellow. However, metallurgists can alter its colour by mixing it with other metals.. Therefore, adding palladium (nickel) gives white gold; adding copper gives it from a red to a rose tinge.

So, when you are buying elegant, classic gold earrings or some pretty heart-shaped ones, you need to know how much gold is in them (the carat) and what it is mixed with (perhaps 62.5% copper) before you can choose.

Body Art

Tiger Face Painting Tips

Tigers are very well-liked animals because of their elegance, agility and power. Children may not see tigers in this light depending on their age and level of understanding of course. Young children see them on TV and they look like little more that big pussy cats and older children, especially in the Developed World, almost certainly do not realize the terror that a stray tiger in the region can instigate.

In spite of that more people like tigers than loathe them. This is one of the factors why the tiger face is very well-liked as a pattern for face painting for children's dos. Face painting has been common with numerous cultures for thousands of years although most individuals would imagine that it is a contemporary phenomenon.

Think of ancient cultures like America's Native Tribes and their war paint. The ancient Celts in northern Europe used woad as war paint and make-up. Aborigine Australians used face paint and so have Asians from India and Pakistan to China and

Japan where the most well-known wearers of face paint are the Geisha girls.

Tigers are in essence Asian animals, so it is no wonder that Asians have revered this huge wild cat for thousands of years and began using it as a style in face painting.

If you want to attempt painting a tiger face onto your child's face, be sure that the paints that you use are safe for purpose and certainly do not contain any lead. However, there are special face painting kits obtainable that should all be trustworthy.

First of all, clean the face of any natural oil and perspiration and then dry it. If the child has long hair, tie it back until you are finished. Some face paints are applied with a damp sponge, so we will go with that procedure for now. First apply a white foundation around the eyes and where a man's beard would be.

Next apply yellow to the centre of the face including the nose but not the tip of the nose. Paint an orange border around the edge of your creation to separate it from the hairline and clothes. Then comes black; applying it with a brush, paint on a few stripes, the whiskers and the tip of the nose. The last step, if desired, is to add a bit of golden glitter to better catch the light.

With a little practice, a tiger face can be applied almost as quickly as the paint dries and you could paint on a number of children at a time, applying say, the white, to as many children as it takes for the first one to dry.

As said above, there are plenty of face painting kits on the market. Look out for Crayola. They provide a cheap kit for about $12 and it comes with paints, brushes, sponges and directions. There are others too. You can remove the tiger face paint with ordinary baby lotion or baby oil on a wad of cotton wool.
I have described the basic 'tiger face', but there are plenty of varieties. look at the Disney cartoon tigers for inspiration or go to the zoo to see how truthful they were at Disney.

Body Art

Airbrush Tanning

Since some people began imagining that a suntanned body makes them look thinner, presumably on the same principle that black clothing makes you look slimmer than white clothing, there has been a dash for instant tans and there is no more instantaneous a tan than to have one painted on. This is known as airbrush tanning.

Airbrush tanning can appeal on different levels. It is fast, you can get any shade you like and there is no risk from UV rays natural or artificial. lots of people are frightened by the stories of skin cancer that they can get by sunbathing or using a tanning bed, so an instantaneous golden bronze colour seems quite an appealing alternative.

The fad for airbrush tanning has spurred the tanning industry to manufacture a vast range of airbrush-look-alike products. There are creams and lotions and even pills that the manufacturers claim will turn your skin an attractive golden bronze. Unfortunately, most of them turn your skin a rather ridiculous shade of orange.

Then there are the home airbrush tanning kits. Real airbrush tanning is the equivalent of having your car resprayed. You can either have it done by a specialist who has professional spraying apparatus or you could go out and purchase twelve cans of your favourite colour car spray paint and do it yourself.

A car sprayed in the former fashion normally looks great, but a car sprayed in the latter manner normally looks dreadful. Well, the same goes for professional salon airbrush tanning and home airbrush tanning. Even amongst professional spray painters some are better than others, so it is best to ask around before you let anyone airbrush you.

So, these are the greatest concerns with airbrush tanning. You cannot do it yourself; you cannot trust a friend to do it for you; it is doubtful whether you can even purchase the right equipment to do it yourself and where do you find a professional whom enough individuals have allowed to practice on them so that he or she is any good?

Because a good airbrush tanner will need the right apparatus and plenty of experience. It is not a trade that can be learned from a book. Airbrush tanning is still a rather new phenomenon, so a decent tanner might be difficult to find outside a big city, but you could try asking the owner of your neighbourhood tanning salon to get one in once a fortnight for those who have booked in advance. A sort of guest appearance.

As with any paint job, the secret to a decent finish is preparation. If you have never been spray-painted before make sure that you prepare yourself properly. Ask your salon to supply you with a list of things that you can do in order to prepare your body in the correct manner.

Preparatory procedures may include shaving and exfoliating but will entail removing all make-up and body oils by showering well. This will give the paint a decent substrate to stick to. The better the preparation you do the better and longer-lasting the airbrush tan - ask any painter and decorator or car sprayer.

Body Art

Some Facts about Tattoos

Tattoos are a sort of man-made scar, that can be coloured at will. Ink is introduced below the skin with a needle where it changes the natural pigmentation of the skin. In olden days, this may have been done with a sharpened feather or a splinter of timber; later, pins and needles were used. Nowadays a tattoo artist uses something that is similar to a road drill, but in miniature.

This tattoo gun has interchangeable needles (one per customer) and can inject ink at the frequency of 2,000 pin pricks a minute. It makes a sound like a dentist's drill. The needle punctures the skin to the required depth and deposits a small amount of ink.

The movement of the needle can be regulated by a small electric motor or it can come from a rope going around a pulley like an old Singer sewing machine, again, just like most dentists' drills. Which sort of machine the tattoo artist operates relies very far on his personal preferences or the item that he learned his trade with.

Disease and infection have always been the greatest

worries when having a tattoo done and that was thousands of years before HIV-AIDS was ever heard of. Even a hundred years ago, an infection in a tattoo on the bicep might mean losing an arm which would have been disastrous for the prosperity of that man and all the members of his family. Being tattooed has always been very risky.

However, even with HIV-AIDS, being tattooed is almost certainly less risky now than it ever has been in history. This is for several factors:

1] tattoo artists and patrons are a lot more aware of the dangers these days

2] tattoo artists require qualifications which means that they have been trained in health and safety awareness

3] tattooing is regulated by the local government's environmental health division in most countries

Therefore, if the customer merely carries out a couple of checks before using a tattoo studio, the risks of serious consequences are fairly negligible. The first thought for most people is the quality of the tattoo and that is obviously very desirable, but the first thought ought to be health and safety. Is the studio clean and is a new needle used for every customer and then thrown away?

Not just the needles need to be sterile and for one use only though. Anything that that needle touches after it has been underneath someone's skin ought to be similarly sterile or disease may be passed through secondary apparatus.

Pain is of secondary importance to most people who go for tattoos. Indeed, some claim that it hurts like the devil and some say that it does not hurt at all. The site of the tattoo and the customer's personal pain threshold play roles here.

However, one thing is sure, a tattoo is an open wound until it heals, so infection can take place after leaving the tattoo parlour as well. That is why it is vital to follow the health and safety advice of the tattooist after you leave his studio.

Body Art

Plastic Surgery Widens Its Scope

Plastic surgery was, until about the turn of the century, always regarded as the exclusive privilege of the rich and famous. It was extremely expensive cosmetic surgery, that only they could afford to pursue.
However, that is no longer the case, and prices have been plummeting.

Many of the middle-class no longer have qualms about getting a nip here and a tuck there, and either paying for it outright or financing it. Part of the reason for this is that the procedures have become more regulated and therefore safer. The staid middle-class, which would not have trusted body-enhancing surgery to foreign hospitals and clinics, have now realised that such plastic surgery manoeuvres carried out abroad, are done so by surgeons, doctors and staff that have been trained to the highest standards.

There is no longer any real need to fear going to Asia, for example, to have a nose job – er, I mean, rhinoplasty, - because the staff involved have the qualifications to work in the West, if they wanted to.

Indeed, it is quite common to see people from the entertainment industry seeking enhancement surgeries and other cosmetic reconstruction surgery sitting in waiting-room seats next to mothers from the suburbs, college students and a growing number of men from a wide variety of ethnic backgrounds. Yes, even men are getting in on the act these days, although that should not really be a surprise as Western men have recently started to take a lot more interest in their appearance.

There is also an obvious demographic shift taking place. Plastic surgery has become a fairly commonplace phenomenon among the middle class of all ethnicities, because the perception that it is exclusively an option for rich, white women is on the decline. People from all walks of life are waking up to the possibility of cosmetic surgery.

It is not uncommon for plastic surgery clinics to offer their patients customized financing packages to cover individual procedures either. The most common procedures for middle-aged women are the tummy tuck, the breast lift (or a breast augmentation with a small breast implant) and the removal of cellulite. It is seen as a quick way of regaining the youthful image that having children stole from them.

Although the cost of commonplace cosmetic surgical procedures has fallen considerably, there are always those who want what is just out of their reach financially. The more cautious of these people save up for their procedures, but others simply finance them and pay for it in with the holiday fund by instalments.

It is important to note that cosmetic plastic surgery used to be quite painful, involving a protracted period of recovery, during which infection was a big risk. However, techniques have vastly improved, as have the medications available to treat and prevent infection. It is now perfectly feasible to have a cosmetic operation done while on holiday, and still enjoy oneself; or to have the operation carried out on a Saturday morning, and be back in work on Monday!

If cosmetic plastic surgery is something that you long to try, just search online; do your research; take advice; and go for it!

Body Art

What Are Bags Under Your Eyes?

Bags under your eyes are traditionally associated with a lack of sleep, but the fact is that some people are more prone to them that others. Some of this has to do with lack of sleep, fair enough, but other reasons are age, skin sort and bone structure.

Therefore, if you start getting bags under your eyes all of a sudden, then you can presume that the problem is because of recent events, but if you just find that the bags are becoming more and more obvious as you become older, then the reason might be more basic.

Numerous people, particularly women, spend time each day of their adult life looking after the skin under their eyes, because they know that that region of their face is the most scrutinized by friends and strangers alike. People are conscious that their eyes are mirrors of their feelings (or even souls) and they would like those mirrors to be set in as attractive frames as possible.

The fact is that for the majority of younger people, the reason for bags under the eyes is as simple as lack of sleep. However, it is the cause of the lack of sleep that ought to be the main anxiety.

If it is merely because they have young babies, then that is par for the course or if it is because of partying all night, the remedy is simple, but if it is because they are worrying all night then that is something else. The cause for the worry has to be sorted out.

Illness is another cause for getting ugly, sagging skin under your eyes and then it is a question of going to the doctor. Sleeping disorders such as sleep apnoea and insomnia also come into this category, but doctors can help here too.

There are thousands or treatments for loose skin under your eyes, which come about as a result of weakening facial skin muscles, which usually happens through age. Some individuals use expensive skin creams and others opt to use more traditional cures. However, both the expensive creams and the traditional remedies usually rely on the use of astringents.

I cannot profess to know which are the best creams, but I can list a few of the time-honoured remedies for loose skin under your eyes. Many individuals try used tea bags, slices of cucumber or cold eye covers like wet cotton wool that has been kept in the fridge or even the freezer.

Still other people prefer an immediate and more permanent remedy for the bags under their eyes and opt for surgery. This form of surgery is not as radical as having a full face lift but it works in a similar manner. A person who undergoes tucks under the eyes will have black eyes for a short time and a little discomfort at first, but the improvement will last for years.

Some people opt to have this type of surgery done 'while on holiday' somewhere, so that none of their friends notice that they have black eyes for a couple of days. The same sort of procedure can remove heavy-looking, low-hanging eyelids.

Owen Jones

Contact Details

Facebook: AngunJones
Twitter: @owen_author
Blog: Megan Publishing Services

This book is part of the 'How to...' series of 125 manuals by Owen Jones.
Links to the whole series in many languages can be found on:
Megan Publishing Services
https://meganthemisconception.com

www.ingramcontent.com/pod-product-compliance
Ingram Content Group UK Ltd.
Pitfield, Milton Keynes, MK11 3LW, UK
UKHW021646190726
13853UKWH00001B/77